S HUGHLEY

HEALTHY LIVING

Live Long Finish Strong

First edition

This book was professionally typeset on Reedsy.
Find out more at reedsy.com

Contents

INTRODUCTION TO HEALTHY LIVING

Hey, fellow seekers of a healthier life! In the midst of life's whirlwind filled with sedentary habits, less-than-ideal diets, and stress levels off the charts, the call to take charge of our well-being has never been louder. This guide is your compass, designed to navigate the maze of adopting a healthier lifestyle. It's not just about pumping iron; it's about embracing a full-on, holistic approach. Think beyond just the gym—this is a journey into the realms of mental and spiritual well-being. From the power-packed trio of exercise, diet, and rest to stress-relieving techniques and most importantly, meditation and prayer, we're discussing it all. So, gear up for an adventure where small, intentional choices lead to a life that's not just healthier but more resilient, fulfilling, and uniquely yours. Let's get started on this journey to a healthier, happier you!

In this fast paced world where our days fly by faster than our minds can comprehend, we are faced with an unprecedented challenge to literally fight for our health, our minds and our emotions. Every media outlet promotes fast food, soft and sports drinks, desserts packed with sugar sugar sugar and we don't even want to get into the rising cost of food, especially healthy foods. Let's face it, our lives are spent 8, 12, 16 hours

sitting and watching screens of one size or another. We **sit** for hours on end without even getting up to go out and eat (and **sit** some more). We eat our breakfast and lunch at our desks where we continue to stare at screens. Then go home, **sit** at the dinner table and move to **sit** or even worse, lie down because we've eaten too much or we're just plain tired. We fall asleep in the chair or on the sofa, drag ourselves to bed to sleep for a few hours then back into this vicious cycle again.

There are so many benefits to a healthier lifestyle some of which include:

- **Promoting better sleep patterns**. Quality sleep is essential for physical and mental recovery, supporting overall well-being.
- **Building a Stronger Immune System**: Regular exercise and a balanced diet contribute to a robust immune system. This helps the body defend against illnesses and infections more effectively.
- **Helping to manage our body weight.** Combined with proper nutrition and regular exercise, it can prevent weight-related issues and promote a healthy body mass index (BMI).
- **Boost energy levels:** Engaging in regular physical activity and maintaining a nutritious diet can boost energy levels. This increased energy can enhance productivity and overall quality of life.
- **Improve cognitive function:** Physical activity is associated with improved cognitive function and a lower risk of cognitive decline as individuals age. It can positively impact memory, attention, and problem-solving skills.
- **Better Emotional Well-being:** A healthy lifestyle can posi-

tively influence emotional well-being. This includes a sense of accomplishment from achieving fitness goals, improved self-esteem, and a more positive outlook on life.

- **Longevity:** Adopting a healthy lifestyle is linked to increased life expectancy. By taking care of the body and mind, individuals are more likely to enjoy a longer and healthier life.

In summary, a healthy lifestyle contributes to overall well-being by improving physical health, mental health, and longevity. It is a holistic approach that encompasses various aspects of life to achieve a balanced and fulfilling existence. Embarking on a journey toward a healthier life isn't just about counting reps or calories; it's about embracing a holistic perspective. Imagine health not as a checklist but as a symphony, where physical fitness dances with mental clarity and spiritual nourishment. This chapter will guide you through the interconnected dimensions of your well-being, revealing the transformative potential when you view health from a 360-degree angle.

Why are we diving into this world of healthier living? It's not just about avoiding the doctor's office; it's about crafting a life that feels vibrant and fulfilling. The purpose of adopting a healthier lifestyle is really to enhance your overall quality of life. From preventing health issues to boosting vitality, this is your roadmap to understanding why each positive choice you make is a crucial step toward a brighter, more energized future.

Feeling overwhelmed? Fear not! This guide is your motivational boost, reminding you that **you** hold the power to transform your life. ***It's not about drastic changes but about small, intentional***

choices. From setting realistic goals to overcoming obstacles, this book is your toolkit for empowerment. It's about embracing change not as a burden but as an opportunity to become the healthiest, happiest version of yourself.

Now, let's talk about the road ahead. First we want to lay out the journey to a healthier lifestyle. Each chapter is a doorway, leading you through the essentials of exercise, the wisdom of a balanced diet, the importance of rest, stress management techniques, and the soul-nurturing practices of meditation and prayer. So, fasten your seatbelt; we're navigating this path together, one chapter at a time.

CHAPTER ONE - MEDITATION AND PRAYER

One of the first and most important ingredients for healthy living is prayer and meditation. 15 minutes first thing in the morning will have a direct influence on how your day will unfold. You cannot control **what** happens but you can control **how** you will respond. These 15 minutes will help you get to your "peace" and you will have much greater success navigating whatever challenges your day may bring.

For individuals who practice Christianity, prayer holds profound importance as a foundation for a healthy and spiritually enriched life. Beyond its religious significance, prayer serves as a direct connection with God, fostering a deep sense of faith, trust, and surrender. The act of prayer is interwoven with the Christian belief in seeking guidance, finding strength in times of adversity, and expressing gratitude for blessings received. Additionally, the practice of prayer aligns with biblical teachings and study, emphasizing the importance of prayer for inner peace, mental clarity, and a strengthened relationship with God. In essence, prayer becomes not only a spiritual discipline but also a transformative force that contributes to the holistic well-being of individuals in their Christian journey.

For those who practice other religions or no religion at all, prayer and meditation foster a sense of connection, purpose and inner peace. Engaging in prayer provides a moment of reflection, allowing individuals to express gratitude, seek guidance, and find solace in times of difficulty. The act of prayer is intertwined with a sense of hope and resilience, offering a spiritual anchor in the face of life's challenges. Moreover, the intentional focus on prayer and meditation instills a sense of mindfulness, promoting mental clarity and reducing stress. This holistic approach to well-being underscores the significance of prayer and meditation as a major component of a healthy and balanced life.

Meditation and prayer are powerful tools for stress reduction, allowing individuals to tap into a state of deep relaxation. They involve focusing on the present moment as the mind gradually releases the grip on stressors. The calming effect triggers the body's relaxation response, lowering cortisol levels and promoting a sense of tranquility.

Meditation contributes significantly to emotional well-being by fostering self-awareness and emotional regulation. Through mindfulness practices, individuals develop the ability to observe their thoughts and emotions without becoming overwhelmed by them. This heightened self-awareness enables a more intentional response to emotional triggers, leading to improved emotional resilience and a greater sense of emotional balance.

A key component of meditation is mindfulness, which involves cultivating a non-judgmental awareness of the present moment. This heightened state of mindfulness has a positive impact on mental health by reducing rumination and overthinking. By staying present and fully engaging in the current experience, individuals can break free from the cycle of repetitive, negative thoughts, promoting a more positive and balanced mental state.

Establishing a regular prayer and meditation practice means setting a consistent schedule. Set aside a dedicated time each day for meditation or prayer to establish a routine. Wear loose clothes and sit in a comfortable position. You need a quiet space to create a peaceful and quiet environment. Start with short sessions of five to ten minutes each day and gradually increase the duration as your comfort level increases. Be patient. Be persistent. Be faithful, knowing you will find a greater sense of peace as you progress and your days will begin with a greater confidence in your ability to accomplish so much more than you ever have experienced.

Both meditation and prayer contribute to a sense of spiritual well-being, fostering a connection with one's inner self or higher power. Both practices involve setting positive intentions, whether it's cultivating compassion, gratitude, or inner peace. Meditation and prayer provide opportunities for self-reflection, allowing individuals to gain insight into their thoughts, emotions, and beliefs. They help us cope with stressful situations and allow us to regain composure and perspective. Also, consider winding down the day with prayer to promote relaxation and restful sleep.

CHAPTER TWO - EXERCISE

Regular physical activity is the cornerstone of a healthy lifestyle, offering a multitude of benefits for both the body and mind. Engaging in consistent exercise not only enhances cardiovascular health, strengthens muscles, and improves flexibility but also plays a crucial role in weight management. Beyond the physical, it releases endorphins, the body's natural mood boosters, promoting mental well-being and reducing stress. The habit of regular activity is a powerful investment in long-term health, fostering resilience, and contributing to an overall sense of vitality and balance in daily life.

Cardiovascular Benefits - Embarking on a regular cardiovascular exercise routine, whether through brisk walks, jogging, cycling, or dancing (which I love the most), promises so many health benefits. Your heart becomes more robust, efficiently pumping blood throughout your body. Blood pressure takes a dip, offering a protective shield against hypertension. The entire circulatory system gets a tune-up, improving oxygen flow and nutrient delivery to every nook and cranny. Picture this not just as a workout but as a daily investment in a heart that beats stronger, propelling you toward a life full of energy .Exercise contributes to overall cardiovascular fitness, enhancing the efficiency of your heart and lungs. This improved cardiac function means your heart can pump more blood with each beat, providing the body with the necessary oxygen and nutrients. **Cardiovascular benefits include:**

   a. Improved heart health: Regular exercise strengthens the heart, reducing the risk of heart disease and improving overall cardiovascular function.

   b. Lower blood pressure: Exercise helps maintain healthy blood pressure levels, reducing strain on the heart and arteries.

   c. Enhanced blood circulation: Physical activity promotes efficient blood flow, ensuring oxygen and nutrients reach all parts of the body.

Weight Management - Incorporating regular exercise into your routine is a key player in effective weight management. Beyond burning calories, physical activity revs up your metabolism and builds lean muscle, contributing to a healthier body composition. It's not just about shedding pounds; it's about cultivating a sustainable and active lifestyle. Whether it's a brisk walk, a workout session, or a dance class, staying active keeps your weight in check while promoting overall well-being. Making exercise a consistent part of your routine becomes a supportive ally in the journey toward maintaining a healthy weight. **Weight management Benefits include:**

   a. Caloric expenditure: Exercise aids in burning calories, contributing to weight loss and maintenance.

   b. Boosted metabolism: Regular physical activity helps maintain a healthy metabolism, facilitating weight control.

   c. Muscle toning: Strength training exercises build lean muscle mass, supporting a toned and fit appearance.

Improved muscle strength and flexibility - Regular exercise brings a dynamic duo to the table: improved muscle strength and flexibility. Engaging in activities that challenge your muscles, such as resistance training or yoga, not only helps you build strength but also enhances your range of motion. This tag team is vital for daily activities, from lifting groceries to reaching high shelves. Improved muscle strength provides stability, while increased flexibility ensures your body moves with ease. Together, they contribute to better overall mobility, reducing the risk of injuries and supporting a more agile and resilient you. A strong, flexible body is your ticket to a life filled with agility and grace. **Improved muscle strength and flexibility benefits include:**

    a. **Increased strength**: Resistance training enhances muscle strength, improving overall functional abilities.

    b. **Enhanced flexibility:** Stretching exercises promote flexibility, reducing the risk of injuries and enhancing range of motion.

    c. **Better posture and balance:** Regular exercise contributes to improved posture and balance, reducing the likelihood of falls and injuries

Types of Exercises - No need to confine yourself to a monotonous exercise routine. I encourage you to explore the diverse spectrum of exercises. Dive into aerobic activities like running or swimming (which I love the most), bicycling for heart-pounding joy. Unleash the power of strength training with bodyweight exercises or weights. For a zen-like experience, embrace flexibility exercises stretching the whole body, promoting suppleness in both body and mind. The key is finding what sparks your joy, turning each workout into a celebration of movement.

Weekly Exercise Recommendations - Crafting a workout routine is like finding the right rhythm for your body. Aim for at least 150 minutes of moderate-intensity aerobic exercise weekly, or half that if the intensity kicks up a notch. Don't forget the strength training duet—two sessions per week will do wonders. This isn't about extremes; it's about finding a groove that syncs with your lifestyle, ensuring you dance through life with strength and vitality. Regular exercise is one of the best things you can do for your health. It has many benefits. It can improve your overall health and fitness and reduce your risk for many chronic diseases.To get the most benefit, *NIH: National Heart, Lung, and Blood Institute* suggests the following:

For adults: Get at least 150 minutes of moderate-intensity or 75 minutes of vigorous-intensity aerobic physical activity each week. Or you could do a combination of the two: Try to spread your physical activity out over several days of the week. That's better than trying to do it all in one or two days. You should try not to do vigorous intense workouts two days in a row. Our bodies need rest in between.

- Some days you may not have long blocks of time to do physical activity. You can try splitting it up into segments of ten minutes or more.
- Aerobic activities include walking fast, jogging, swimming, and biking
- Moderate intensity means that while you are doing that activity, you should be able to say a few words in a row but not sing
- Vigorous intensity means that while you are doing that activity, you won't be able to say more than a few words

without stopping for a breath

Also, do strengthening activities at least twice per week.:

- Strengthening activities include lifting weights, working with exercise bands, and doing sit-ups and push ups
- Choose activities that work all the different parts of the body – your legs, hips, back, chest, stomach, shoulders, and arms. You should repeat exercises for each muscle group 3 repetitions of 10 counts.

Also, try to get each of these at least 3 days a week: vigorous-intensity aerobic activity, muscle-strengthening activity, and bone-strengthening activity.:

- Vigorous-intensity aerobic activities include running, doing jumping jacks, and fast swimming
- Muscle-strengthening activities include playing on play-ground equipment, playing tug-of-war, and doing pushups and pull-ups
- Bone-strengthening activities include hopping, skipping, doing jumping jacks, playing volleyball, and working with resistance bands

Older adults, pregnant women, and people who have special health needs should check with their health care provider on how much physical activity they should get and what types of activities they should do.

Exercise tips: People who are trying to lose weight may need to get more physical activity. They also need to adjust their diet, so they are burning more calories than they eat and drink. If you have been inactive, you may need to start slowly. You can keep adding more gradually. The more you can do, the better. But try not to feel overwhelmed, and do what you can. Getting some physical activity is always better than getting none.

Remember to warm up before stretching and perform these exercises regularly to improve and maintain flexibility. If you have any existing health conditions, it's advisable to consult with a healthcare professional or fitness expert before starting a new exercise routine.

STAY MOTIVATED - Setting realistic goals, both short-term and long-term, keeps the fire alive. Find activities that spark joy, making each workout a delightful experience. Embrace variety; changing up your routine prevents monotony. Overcoming obstacles is part of the journey, so don't be too hard on yourself. Track your progress; every step is a victory. With these motivational notes, you'll not only initiate but sustain your fitness journey, ensuring a healthier, happier you.

CHAPTER THREE - DIET

A balanced and nutritious diet serves as the fundamental fuel that powers a healthier lifestyle. Each bite is an opportunity to provide the body with a wide variety of essential nutrients, including vitamins, minerals, proteins, and complex carbohydrates. These nutrients play a crucial role in supporting the body's various functions, from building a strong immune system to supporting cell repair and growth. Eating nutrient-packed foods helps your body get everything it needs to work well, giving you more energy and making you feel healthier overall.

Beyond nourishment, a balanced diet plays a crucial role in weight management and maintaining satisfaction. Consuming a variety of foods in the right proportions helps regulate calorie intake and prevents overeating. Foods rich in fiber, such as fruits, vegetables, and whole grains, contribute to a feeling of fullness, reducing the likelihood of unhealthy snacking. Moreover, a balanced diet helps strike the right balance of macronutrients, ensuring that the body receives an appropriate mix of carbohydrates, proteins, and fats, essential for sustained energy and healthy metabolic function.

The choices made at our dining table will have great implications for long-term health. A balanced and nutritious diet is a powerful weapon against various health conditions, including heart disease, diabetes, and certain cancers. Antioxidant-rich fruits and vegetables combat oxidative stress, while foods low in saturated fats contribute to heart health. The long-term effect of a healthy diet extends far beyond immediate well-being, but also contributes to longevity and reduces the risk of chronic diseases. By viewing each meal as an opportunity to build and strengthen the body's defenses, you will proactively invest in your long-term health and well-being.

Nutrient-rich foods are like powerhouse champions for your body, providing an abundance of essential vitamins, minerals, and other goodies that keep everything running smoothly. Think of colorful fruits and veggies, whole grains, lean proteins, and dairy or dairy alternatives – these foods are the real MVPs. They offer a variety of nutrients that support your immune system, help your bones and muscles stay strong, and give you the energy to tackle your day. Incorporating nutrient-rich foods into your diet isn't just about eating; it's about nourishing your body with the good stuff it needs to thrive. So, load up your plate with a rainbow of wholesome foods and let your body revel in the nutrient-packed goodness!

NUTRIENT-RICH FOODS

a. Whole grains: A whole grain is a grain of any cereal and pseudocereal that contains the endosperm, germ, and bran, in contrast to refined grains, which retain only the endosperm. As part of a general healthy diet, consumption of whole grains is associated with lower risk of several diseases. Refined grains have been milled, a process that removes the bran and germ. This is done to give grains a finer texture and improve their shelf life. Choose whole grains over refined grains for higher fiber content and essential nutrients. Some whole-grain examples are **whole-wheat flour, bulgur (cracked wheat), oatmeal, and brown rice, barley, farro, millet, quinoa, black rice, brown rice and red rice.**

b. Fruits and vegetables: Having a colorful variety of fruits and vegetables in your diet is like giving your body a nutrition party. Each fruit and veggie brings its unique set of vitamins, minerals, and antioxidants, offering a fantastic range of health benefits so aim for a variety of colorful fruits. Fruits and vegetables are rich in many nutrients such as potassium, folate and vitamins A and C. From the vibrant antioxidants in berries to the bone-strengthening power of leafy greens, this diverse mix supports your immune system, boosts energy levels, and keeps your body happy and strong. It's not just about preventing boredom on your plate; it's about providing your body with a symphony of nutrients that work together to keep you feeling your best. So, pile on the colors, mix up your options, and let the variety of fruits and veggies turn your meals into a nutritional celebration for your overall well-being. Be sure to check the sugar content in fruit, especially fruit juices. Some fruit have a much higher sugar content than others and we're trying to avoid that overload of sugar..

c. Lean proteins: Opting for lean meats is like giving your body a health upgrade. These meats, like skinless poultry, fish, bison or lean cuts of beef or pork, pack a punch of protein without the excess saturated fats found in their fattier counterparts. Protein is your body's superhero, supporting muscle growth, repair, and overall strength. By choosing lean meats, you're not only fueling your muscles but also keeping your heart happy and healthy.

The lower fat content means you're getting a nutrient-rich package without the added baggage of excessive calories or cholesterol. It's a smart choice for those looking to maintain a healthy weight, support muscle health, and keep their overall well-being in top shape. So, next time you're at the butcher's counter, think lean for a delicious and health-conscious meal.

Diversifying your protein sources with options like tofu or beans is like broadening the nutritional palette for your body. Tofu, a plant-based protein, brings not just protein but also a dose of heart-healthy fats and minerals. Beans, whether black, kidney, or chickpeas, deliver a protein punch along with fiber, aiding digestion and keeping you full. By incorporating these alternatives, you're not only offering your body a break from animal proteins but also tapping into a variety of essential nutrients. Plus, these plant-based options are often lower in saturated fats, making them a heart-smart choice. Whether you're exploring a vegetarian lifestyle or just aiming for a well-rounded diet, adding tofu, beans, and similar sources to your plate ensures you're meeting your protein needs while embracing the health perks of plant-based eating.

 d. **Healthy fats**: Embracing healthy fats in your diet is like giving your body a boost of nutritional goodness. Sources like avocados, nuts, seeds, and olive oil are rich in unsaturated fats (monounsaturated and polyunsaturated), which are known to promote heart health. These fats contribute to a balanced lipid profile, supporting good cholesterol levels while keeping bad cholesterol in check. Healthy fats are not just a fuel source; they also aid in the absorption of fat-soluble vitamins like A, D, E, and K, ensuring your body reaps the full benefits of these nutrients. Including these fats in your diet can also help with helping you feel full, making you feel satisfied and less likely to overeat. So, rather than fearing fats, choosing the right kinds can be a flavorful and essential part of a well-rounded, healthy eating plan.

Portion Control: Portion control is the guiding principle that empowers individuals to manage their food intake wisely. It's not about restrictive diets or denying yourself your favorite foods; instead, it's a mindful approach to understanding how much your body needs. By being conscious of portion sizes, you can maintain a healthy weight, support digestion, and regulate energy levels.

Portion control encourages:

- a balanced relationship with food
- prevents overeating and
- promotes a greater awareness of hunger and fullness cues

It's a practical strategy that allows individuals to enjoy a variety of foods while ensuring that each meal is a well-balanced and satisfying experience. Through the simple yet impact practice of portion control, individuals can take charge of their nutrition, fostering a healthier and more mindful approach to eating.

Hydration – Drink water, water, water…: Hydration is the unsung hero of well–being, playing a crucial role in maintaining overall health. Just as our bodies rely on various systems to function optimally, they equally depend on an adequate supply of water. Sufficient hydration supports digestion, nutrient absorption, and temperature regulation. Beyond quenching our thirst, water is a fundamental building block for cellular activities and metabolic processes. It revitalizes our skin, boosts cognitive function, and aids in flushing out toxins. In essence, staying properly hydrated isn't just about satisfying a basic need; it's a cornerstone of a thriving and energized life. So, sip by sip, hydrate your way to vitality, giving your body the essential fluid foundation it needs to perform at its best.

Food groups and their role in a healthy diet
  1. Fruits and vegetables
  a. **Benefits**: Rich in vitamins, minerals, fiber, and antioxidants, promoting overall health and reducing the risk of chronic diseases.
  b. **Recommended servings**: Aim for a variety of colors and at least 5 servings per day.

  2. Whole grains
  a. **Benefits**: Provide essential nutrients, fiber, and sustained energy, supporting heart health and weight management.
  b. **Examples**: Brown rice, quinoa, whole wheat, oats.

  3. Lean proteins

   a. Benefits: Essential for muscle repair, immune function, and overall growth and development.

   b. Examples: Chicken, turkey, fish, beans, lentils, tofu.

4. Healthy fats

   a. Benefits: Support brain function, hormone production, and overall cellular health.

   b. Examples: Avocado, olive oil, nuts, seeds, fatty fish.

C. Meal planning and Preparation Tips

Understanding the role of food groups is another key to unlocking the secret for a healthy and balanced diet. Each food group brings a unique set of nutrients, contributing to overall well-being. Fruits and vegetables, rich in vitamins, minerals, and fiber, are the colorful champions that support immune function and digestive health. Whole grains, the steadfast foundation, provide complex carbohydrates for sustained energy and essential nutrients. Lean proteins, found in sources like skinless poultry, fish, and legumes, are the building blocks for muscle repair and growth. Dairy or dairy alternatives offer calcium for strong bones and teeth. Healthy fats, sourced from avocados, nuts, and olive oil, contribute to heart health and aid in nutrient absorption. By incorporating a variety of foods from these groups, individuals can create a symphony of nutrients, ensuring that their diet is a harmonious blend of flavors and health benefits.

Some helpful tips:

   1. Plan meals in advance: Outline a weekly menu to ensure a balanced and varied diet. Don't be afraid to be creative. Mix and match different combinations to ensure both good health and tasty meals. A good menu will help you shop for groceries and keep you from just putting "junk food" in your shopping basket.

2. Cook at home: Prepare meals at home using fresh ingredients to have control over portion sizes and ingredients. Since you have no control over what happens in a restaurant kitchen, the safest way to ensure the ingredients in your meal is to prepare it at home. There are so many incredibly delicious recipes to choose from online.

3. Keep healthy snacks available: Have nutritious snacks readily available to avoid reaching for unhealthy options during moments of hunger. If it's not in your house, you can't reach for it when you want something to snack on... so don't stock up with the "junk food" in your pantry. Great snacks include nuts, raw carrots and celery. Nut butters and hummus are delicious on rice crackers, veggies and fruit.

4. Read food labels: Be aware of nutritional content and ingredients to make informed choices while shopping. You don't realize how much added sugar and sodium (salt) are added to foods. Reading the labels is so important on your journey to a healthy diet.

5. Practice mindful eating: Slow down, savor each bite, and pay attention to hunger and fullness cues for a healthier relationship with food. According to studies including ***Healthline.com*** food should be chewed about **32 times**, foods that are harder to chew, such as steak and nuts may need up to **40 chews** per mouthful. For foods that are softer such as mashed potato and watermelon you can get away with chewing just **5-10 times. So chew your food to help aid in good digestion.**

CHAPTER FOUR - REST

Rest is the unsung hero in the narrative of a healthy lifestyle, often underestimated but profoundly crucial. In a world that glorifies constant productivity, embracing adequate rest is a cornerstone of overall well-being. Quality sleep allows the body to repair and regenerate, supporting optimal physical and mental function. It's during restful moments that muscles recover, immune function strengthens, and the mind processes and consolidates information. Beyond the physical realm, mental and emotional well-being find solace in rest, reducing stress and enhancing resilience. Recognizing the significance of rest is not a luxury but a vital component of a balanced life. By prioritizing sufficient and quality rest, individuals can unlock the door to enhanced energy, improved mood, and sustained vitality, creating a robust foundation for a truly healthy lifestyle.

The National Sleep Foundation provides general sleep duration recommendations for different age groups. According to their guidelines:

- Adults (18-64 years old): 7-9 hours of sleep per night
- Older Adults (65 years and older): 7-8 hours of sleep per night

It's important to note that individual sleep needs may vary, and factors such as overall health, stress levels, and lifestyle can influence the ideal amount of sleep for a person. It's advisable to pay attention to your body's signals and adjust your sleep routine accordingly to ensure optimal well-being.

Impact on Physical Health – Cellular Repair & Hormone regulation

- **During sleep, the body undergoes essential repair processes, promoting overall cellular health.**
- **Adequate sleep supports the regulation of hormones related to stress growth and appetite.**
- **Quality sleep enhances the immune system's ability to defend against infections and illnesses.**

Adequate and quality sleep plays a pivotal role in maintaining and enhancing physical health. During the sleep cycle, the body undergoes essential processes that contribute to overall well-being. Muscles repair and grow, tissues heal, and the immune system strengthens.

Chronic sleep deprivation, on the other hand, has been linked to various adverse physical effects. It can weaken the immune system, making the body more susceptible to illnesses. Additionally, insufficient sleep is associated with an increased risk of conditions such as obesity, diabetes, and cardiovascular diseases.

Beyond the tangible, the impact of sleep on physical health extends to daily functionality – a well-rested body is more alert, focused, and capable of performing at its peak. Prioritizing sufficient and quality sleep is not just a luxury but a fundamental investment in maintaining and optimizing physical health.

Influences on Mental well-being:

- **Sleep is crucial for cognitive functions such as memory consolidation, learning and problem solving.**
- **Adequate sleep also contributes to better emotional resilience and the ability to cope with stress.**
- **Finally, quality sleep improves focus, concentration and overall mental clarity**

Tips for improving sleep habits

1. Consistent sleep schedule

a. Establish a regular bedtime and wake-up time, even on weekends.

b. Avoid drastic changes in sleep patterns to regulate the body's internal clock.

2. Creating a comfortable sleep environment

a. Optimal sleep conditions: Keep the bedroom dark, quiet, and cool for an ideal sleep environment.

b. Comfortable mattress and pillows: Invest in a comfortable mattress and pillows to support proper alignment and reduce discomfort.

3. Limiting screen time before bed

a. Blue light impact: Reduce exposure to electronic devices emitting blue light, as it can interfere with the production of sleep-inducing hormones.

b. Establish a technology-free zone at least 30 minutes before bedtime to promote relaxation.

CHAPTER V. - STRESS MANAGEMENT

Stress is called the "Silent Killer". Chronic stress isn't just mental strain; it's a silent health menace. Prolonged stress triggers harmful hormones like cortisol, which, in excess, can disrupt the immune system, elevate blood pressure, and contribute to inflammation. This physiological turmoil raises the risk of illnesses and worsens conditions like heart disease. Beyond physical harm, chronic stress takes a toll on mental well–being, contributing to anxiety, depression and insomnia, creating a vicious cycle that further compromises overall health. Recognizing and managing stress is crucial to preserving a healthy lifestyle, striking a balance between mind and body.

Stress Reduction Techniques

1. Prayer and meditation
   a. Deep breathing: Practice deep breathing exercises to calm the nervous system and reduce stress. A simple deep breathing exercise is the 4–7–8 technique:

- Sit comfortably or lie down.
- Close your eyes and take a deep breath in through your nose, counting to four.

- Hold your breath for a count of seven.
- Exhale completely through your mouth, counting to eight.
- Repeat this cycle for a few rounds, gradually extending the counts as you become more comfortable.

This technique can help calm the nervous system, reduce stress, and promote relaxation.

b. Meditation practices: Incorporate mindfulness meditation or guided meditation sessions to promote relaxation.

2. Other deep breathing exercises

a. Diaphragmatic breathing: Engage in deep, diaphragmatic breaths to activate the body's relaxation response. Diaphragmatic breathing, also known as abdominal or deep breathing, involves engaging the diaphragm muscle for more efficient and calming breaths. To practice, inhale deeply through your nose, allowing your diaphragm to expand, then exhale slowly through your mouth. This technique promotes relaxation, reduces stress, and enhances overall respiratory function.

b. Box breathing: Inhale, hold, exhale, and pause for equal durations to enhance relaxation.Box breathing, also known as square breathing, involves inhaling, holding the breath, exhaling, and pausing in a rhythmic four-count pattern. This method is effective for calming the nervous system and promoting a sense of focus and relaxation.

3. Time management strategies

Effective time management is a cornerstone of productivity.

Strategies like prioritizing tasks, breaking them into smaller steps, and setting realistic deadlines can enhance efficiency. Creating to-do lists, utilizing productivity tools, and minimizing multitasking also contribute to better time utilization. Additionally, periodic breaks and dedicating specific time blocks to different activities help maintain focus and prevent burnout. By adopting these time management strategies, individuals can navigate their responsibilities more effectively, ensuring a balanced and productive use of their time.

a. **Prioritize tasks:** Identify and prioritize tasks to manage workload effectively.

b. **Create to-do lists:** We all need order to maximize time and efficiencies

c. **Break tasks into smaller steps**: Breaking down tasks into manageable steps reduces feelings of being overwhelmed.

d. **Take Breaks** - Scheduled breaks every 2 hours are a necessity to maximize productivity. Stand up, walk around, stretch and focus on something other than what we are working on.

4. Incorporating leisure and recreational activities for stress relief

Incorporating leisure and recreational activities into your routine is a powerful stress-relief strategy. Whether it's a brisk walk in nature, engaging in a favorite hobby, or simply taking time for relaxation, these activities provide a mental reset. They not only offer a welcome break from daily stressors but also contribute to improved mood, enhanced creativity, and an overall sense of well-being. These might include:

1. Hobbies and interests: Engage in activities that bring joy and relaxation, whether it's reading, painting, or spending time in nature.

2. Physical activity: Exercise is not only beneficial for physical health but also an effective stress reliever.

3. Social connections: Maintain positive social connections with friends and family for emotional support and stress reduction.

CONCLUSION

In conclusion, healthy living is a multifaceted journey encompassing key components such as regular exercise, a balanced and nutritious diet, sufficient rest, stress management, and mindful practices like meditation and prayer. By prioritizing these elements, individuals can foster physical well-being, mental resilience, and a harmonious connection between mind, body, and spirit. Small, intentional choices made daily contribute to a healthier, more resilient, and fulfilling life. It's not about perfection but the continuous commitment to embracing positive changes, creating a sustainable and personalized path toward holistic well-being.

1.Practice the integration of lifestyle practices for overall well-being

Implementing the integration of lifestyle practices is like assembling a toolkit for overall well-being. It's about blending good habits into our daily lives—like eating nutritious foods, staying active, getting enough rest, and finding time for activities that bring joy. These small choices, when woven together, create a fabric of health that supports our bodies, minds, and spirits. So, let's embrace these simple practices, making them a natural part of our routines for a happier and healthier life overall.

Here are actionable steps to incorporate into daily practice:

- **Morning Meditation and Prayer Time:** Start your day with 15 minutes of quiet prayer and meditation. Quieting your mind and focusing on the Blessings of another day filled with opportunities. Be thankful for the people in your life, your good health, your courage and strength to get through another day.
- **Morning Movement:** Continue your day with a burst of energy through a brief morning exercise routine. This can be as simple as a quick jog, stretching, or a few minutes of yoga to wake up your body and mind.
- **Balanced Breakfast:** Fuel your body with a nutritious breakfast that includes a mix of whole grains, fruits, and proteins. This sets a positive tone for the day and provides sustained energy.
- **Hydration Habit:** Make a conscious effort to stay hydrated throughout the day by drinking enough water. Carry a water bottle with you and take sips regularly to maintain optimal hydration levels.
- **Mindful Meals:** Practice mindful eating by savoring each bite, paying attention to flavors and textures. This helps in better digestion and fosters a healthier relationship with food.
- **Active Breaks:** Incorporate short breaks during the day for light physical activity. Whether it's a brisk walk, stretching, or a quick dance, these breaks keep you energized and focused.
- **Digital Detox:** Allocate specific times for a digital detox, lim-

iting screen time and fostering a healthier balance between virtual and real-world interactions.

- **Evening Wind Down:** Establish a calming routine in the evening to signal your body that it's time to wind down. This can include activities like reading, gentle stretching, or practicing relaxation techniques.
- **Quality Sleep**: Prioritize getting 7-9 hours of quality sleep each night. Create a comfortable sleep environment and establish a consistent bedtime routine for better rest.
- **Gratitude Practice:** Dedicate a few moments each day to reflect on things you're grateful for. This simple practice can enhance your overall outlook and mindset.
- **Joyful Activities:** Make time for activities that bring you joy and relaxation, whether it's pursuing a hobby, spending time with loved ones, or enjoying nature. These moments contribute significantly to overall well-being.

2. Gradual changes:

Making gradual changes is like taking small steps toward big improvements. Instead of overwhelming ourselves with drastic transformations, we introduce small, manageable adjustments to our routines. This approach allows us to build new habits steadily, making them more sustainable in the long run. Whether it's adopting a healthier diet, incorporating exercise, or managing stress, the power of gradual change lies in its gentleness. It gives us the time to adapt, learn, and grow, creating a foundation for lasting and positive transformations in our lives.

3. The long-term benefits

Remembering the long-term benefits serves as a motivational compass on our journey to well-being. It's a reminder that the small, positive choices we make today ripple into a healthier and more fulfilling tomorrow. Whether it's the sustained energy from regular exercise, the resilience built through stress management, or the lasting impact of a balanced lifestyle, these long-term benefits become the driving force behind our daily efforts. Embracing these positive changes isn't just for the present; it's an investment in a future where well-being is a constant companion, supporting us on our path to a vibrant and enduring life.

4. Continued Commitment

The benefit of continued commitment to a healthy lifestyle is the assurance of sustained well-being. It's the promise that each positive choice, each exercise, and every mindful moment compounds over time, building a foundation for lasting health. When we stay committed, we cultivate habits that become second nature, promoting physical fitness, mental resilience, and overall vitality. The journey of continued commitment isn't just about short-term gains; it's an ongoing investment in our long-term health and happiness, ensuring a brighter and more energetic future.

5. Reinforcement of the importance of self-care

Prioritizing self-care is like making a crucial investment in our own well-being – a commitment to nurturing our physical, mental, and spiritual health. It's not a luxury but a necessity, akin to putting on your own oxygen mask before assisting others. Regularly assessing our habits ensures we're attuned to our evolving needs. Just as we adjust the course of a ship to reach its destination, making tweaks to our self-care routines allows us to navigate life's challenges with resilience. This ongoing commitment becomes a compass, guiding us towards a balanced and fulfilling life, where we can give our best to ourselves and others.

6. Inspiring a sense of empowerment

Feeling empowered through your choices is like fueling the engine of a lifelong journey towards well-being. Every small decision you make, like eating well or taking time for yourself, adds up to make a big difference in how you feel. It's not about being perfect, but about realizing you have the power to make things better for yourself. This journey is a long-term commitment to feeling strong, happy, and in control of your well-being. So, keep making those positive choices, and you'll see the awesome impact it has on your life.

www.ingramcontent.com/pod-product-compliance
Lightning Source LLC
Chambersburg PA
CBHW050754250726
48662CB00005B/2220